pH BALANCED
FOR LIFE

Earth Clinic Presents...

pH BALANCED FOR LIFE:

The Easiest Way to Alkalize

By Parhatsathid Napatalung
with Bill Thompson

An Earth Clinic Publication

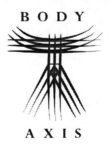

BODY

AXIS

Body Axis, LLC.
Atlanta

DISCLAIMER
The preparation and publication of this book has been undertaken with great care. However, the book is offered for informational purposes only and cannot be taken as a substitute for professional medical prevention, diagnosis, or treatment. Please consult with your physician, pharmacist, or health care provider before taking any home remedies or supplements or following any treatment suggested by anyone within this book. Only your health care provider, personal physician, or pharmacist can provide you with advice on what is safe and effective for your unique needs or diagnose your particular medical history.

Visit us online at:
www.bodyaxis.com
www.earthclinic.com

Printed in the United States of America

FIRST PRINTING: 2012
ISBN-978-0-9828963-7-2

Dedication

Dedicated and with our great thanks to Mr. Parhatsathid Napatalung (aka Ted from Bangkok) and his family, for all his open knowledge, advice and great efforts towards understanding and curing illness and disease.

Table of Contents

ACKNOWLEDGEMENTS

My great and heartfelt thanks to Deirdre Layne, Daniel P. Kray and Earth Clinic for all their wonderful help in advising, promoting and supporting both Ted and myself in this endeavour. And my ultimate and grateful thanks to Ted from Bangkok for all the knowledge that he is freely transmitting concerning his own discoveries and remedies so that other people can achieve good health and lead a happier life. I am still learning and that is always the way it should be.

INTRODUCING MESSIEURS NAPATALUNG AND THOMPSON

The EarthClinic.com online community is now well into its second decade of uncovering and sharing the world's natural secrets for improved and continuing health. For a majority of those years, our most trusted and consistent contributor has been a gentleman by the name of Parhatsathid Napatalung. We have come to know him quite fondly as Ted. A life-long resident of Bangkok, Thailand, Mr. Napatalung is a self-taught expert in natural remedies and collaborative medicine. He maintains impossibly busy online and clinical consultation practices, while still finding time to experiment with increasingly effective healing therapies and passing the lessons of his research on to students locally in Thailand and globally via the Earth Clinic website.

The book you are about to read is the first time Mr. Napatalung's thoughts on a medical subject have been distilled and clarified into a single document. We genuinely hope it will not the last time we get to do so; and by the end of this book, we expect you will be hoping for the same. His knowledge of biochemistry and the nutritional needs of the body for promoting healing and maintaining health have changed lives and the way tens of thousands of us think about our own bodies. Mr. Napatalung's native tongue is Thai, and though he communicates with our online community very effectively in English, his lifetime of study has been dedicated to the intricacies of human health, illness, and healing rather than the clearest expression of the English language. Fortunately, fate also brought a man by the name of Mr. Bill Thompson into the Earth Clinic community of experts.

As you'll soon find out, Bill very naturally became a student of Mr. Napatalung's medical instruction, and through his continued presence on our website subsequently became the acolyte naturally suited to the task of coalescing and clarifying the master's thoughts. In the pages ahead, Bill will introduce himself briefly. What follows thereafter is the voice of Mr. Napatalung as our online community has come to know and love it—only thanks to Mr. Thompson's efforts that voice can now be heard without the distracting fizzle and pop of the long distance call and language differences that heretofore have somewhat stood between us.

We of the EarthClinic.com community were infinitely indebted to both gentlemen for their years of dedication and patient explanations as to how we all, one by one, might set the course of lives back on their intended, healthy tracks. With the publication of this book, the gift of continuing health they deliver unto the world grows immeasurable. We hope you enjoy and are improved by it as much as we so long have been.

Deirdre Layne and the Earth Clinic Team

AUTHOR'S PREFACE

Please Note: From this point on, Mr. Parhatsathid Napata-lung, the originator of these alkalizing protocols, will simply be referred to under the pseudonym of Ted from Bangkok or just as Ted.

This book is a little different from all the other health books on Alkalizing. There are many books on alkalizing – which usually involve using just an alkaline diet – but Ted's alkalizing methods, which are all presented in this book, although fully supporting alkaline and vegetarian diets, is unique and moves a significant step further by using natural body chemicals in the alkalizing protocols to achieve similar, indeed better, results than just using alkalizing diets. This alkalizing protocol also takes another huge step forward in teaching us how to actually monitor our own health state quite cheaply. So all in one book, you will have the means to alkalize your body directly using body friendly alkaline chemicals and diet as well as actually be able to monitor the results. This monitored feedback information allows you to adjust these remedies individually according to your healing needs more accurately as well as telling you what your health status is at any point in time.

My own journey towards Ted's way of healing first occurred over 6 years ago when I realized I had systemic candida. My quality of life had been degenerating and plummeting for about the last 8 to 10 years. But, as a 55-year-old man, I just thought it was old age creeping up on me. But certain problems came to pass that could not be ignored. My candida suddenly became much worse and I had bowel movement only once every week. I was continually bloated, overweight and lethargic with low energy. I suddenly had multiple fungal skin problems and eruptions. I already knew that Nystatin and other anti-fungal remedies would not work very well against systemic candida so I set about finding a proper cure and this is when I stumbled upon Ted's Remedies on the EarthClinic site. I did even more research and validation on his anti-candida remedies and became completely convinced of their efficacy. Then I simply adopted a daily multi-protocol based on Ted's remedies and stuck to this for a whole year without ever deviating -- at the end of which my candida was completely gone and I was healthy again. Along the way – and also using Ted's remedies -- I also cured other problems, which included heart arrhythmia, vertigo, insomnia, hypothyroidism, eczema, psoriasis, tinea cruris, nail fungus and athlete's foot. Early on in the protocols, I also dumped all my gallstones over a month period which I didn't know that I had! As a 62-year-old man, I now feel no different from when I was 35 years old. I have lots of energy, no more aches and pains, healthy heart, memory good and I lost a lot of excess weight easily during this healing process, which also included using Ted's Alkalizing Protocols on a daily basis. The one distinguishing feature in all of Ted's protocols is that his remedies and strategies always address the root cause of any particular disease or problem. My own experience with the medical profession and drugs, regarding the more serious auto-immune diseases, has been disappointing because doctors only ever seem to treat the symptoms. They simply have no clue or firm agreement on what actually causes diseases like Cancer, Obesity, Diabetes, Alzheimer's, Arthritis, Parkinson's, Hepatitis, Allergies, Hyperthyroid, Hypothyroid, Heart Disease, MS, Fibromyalgia etc.

I will always be forever grateful to Ted for opening my own eyes as to what actually becomes possible when you adopt his self-healing alkalizing protocols. In my own riddance of systemic candida and beyond, my thinking has also changed significantly because I have learnt such a great deal about how to cure the root causes of many diseases -- this is the focal point and basis for all of Ted's healing protocols. And one of the main stalwarts of Ted's methods is alkalizing for health, which is fully presented and explained in this book.

The main emphasis and purpose of this book is primarily to convince people of the efficacy and safety of alkalizing regularly using the relatively newer and unique approach of supplementing natural body alkaline chemicals for health and as a remedial tool in the recovery of the body terrain from disease and to present valid reasons why everyone needs to alkalize for health today. The full range of Ted from Bangkok's alkalizing remedies – as well as the newly updated alkalizing remedies – and unique, inexpensive health monitoring methods are also fully presented here.

There are also many important parameters and indicators of health and illness in the body that Ted from Bangkok importantly uses in his assessments of health and disease—these include pH, Conductivity, ORP and Brix measurement factors. These will all be simply explained and discussed in the book in terms of ultimately measuring, tracking and helping the body's *homeostasis* mechanism to recover the body's physiological, chemical and electrical balance – how the body actually achieves its natural and healthy state again through its own balancing mechanisms with help from Alkalizing – after continuously assaulting our own bodies with chemically processed food, medical drugs, poor drinking water, and ingestion of excess halogens, heavy metals and other poisons as well as through a declining share of proper nutrients in our food.

In general and due to all the bad diets, poisons, lack of proper nutrients, pollution and modern stress, the body is perpetually in an unhealthy acid state. The outcome is that the body eventually begins to lose the battle and becomes unhealthy – and this effect can be cumulative over many years – so the body slowly degenerates in health until and because of the effects of a much weakened and stressed immune system, disease and illness take hold with a vengeance

Furthermore, the general concept, approach and reasons for alkalizing the body adhere more to the older and lesser known principles of Prof. Antoine Bechamp and his Terrain or Cellular Theory than to the principles of Pasteur's Germ Theory, so staunchly adhered to by today's allopathic community.

Pasteur more or less defined his approach as:

One Disease → One Germ → One Cure

This is the Germ Theory's main emphasis and basis, which has given rise to its prime method of treatment in using synthetic drugs. Overkill with said drugs results in collateral body damage from side-effects of their attack on the pathogenic germs with consequent suppression of the immune system, further weakening the body terrain—especially in their treatment of the more serious auto-immune diseases like Cancer, Hepatitis C, Hyperthyroidism, Leukemia etc. The Germ Theory originally maintained that pathogens, like bacteria, viruses and fungi, were *monomorphic**, only ever having one form, and this theory also casually assumed that the human body was more or less perfect in form and completely sterile from germs, which could only ever attack the body from the outside.

Antoine Bechamp's somewhat contrary Terrain or Cellular Theory maintained that, above all, the health of the body must be maintained at all costs and that the prime cause of disease was, for the greater part, due to both a weakened body terrain and a weakened immune system. He maintained that dangerous pathogens continuously inhabit and exist in our bodies, acting as friendlier symbionts in our bodies when we are healthy. In other words, our inner pathogens are most adequately and completely suppressed by a healthy body. Current research in fact confirms that the number of good and bad microbes that exist in just our own intestines, is vastly greater than the sum total of actual cells in our own bodies. Dangerous bacteria such as H. Pylori and E. Coli always co-exist with friendly bacteria -- to some degree -- in everyone's intestines and it is only the health of our intestines as well as the strength of our immune system that suppresses their spread and conversion to more virulent pathogenic forms. Similarly, cancer cells are formed in our bodies every single day and it is only through the health and goodness of our own body's defenses that these cancer cells are able to be successfully suppressed or removed. The real point here is essentially a chicken or egg argument – does a pathogen enter our "perfectly sterile and pure body" and then we become ill, thus causing a failure of our immune system to cope (Germ Theory) or does the degeneration of our body's health state and immune system happen first (Terrain Theory) due to a bad diet and lifestyle, such that our inner and outer pathogen(s) are now able to achieve an easy foothold, leading to pathogen dominance and virulence within the body? Both the evidence and common sense would tend to suggest that the latter is true.

So when our bodies become unhealthy and weakened through bad diet, toxins or for whatever reasons, then these friendly symbionts would quite naturally change in their structure and function to swiftly adapt themselves according to the sickness or bad health state of the inner body environment – by a process called *pleomorphism* [see footnote]-- and so these pathogens are then able to change into dangerous parasitic forms or even change themselves into a completely different pathogenic forms, which might then become dangerous and virulent within the human body, thereby causing severe disease and illness. These same principles must also apply with any invasion by a pathogen from outside the body. Simply put, a healthy body terrain with a strong immune system should easily be able to prevent most serious disease and illnesses from arising in the human body.

So the short and simple description of Alkalizing is that it is simply a way of supplementing the body with alkaline nutrients whose effect is to greatly aid body homeostasis (as well as satisfying many other parameters) in its difficult achievement of constant health within our own modern world and lifestyles.

The explanations in this book are deliberately kept as simple as possible in order to be more easily and clearly understood. But if the reader wishes to further pursue this subject in greater depth and scientific detail, then you should access the Resource Appendix in the end chapter for more research information on Alkalizing. This miscellaneous section provides definitions and links to research and book references as further proof of the necessity, safety and efficacy of alkalizing the body.

Furthermore, although I have written this book, the ideas contained herein are all derived from Ted from Bangkok's successful use and experiences of using these alkalizing protocols. I therefore must make the point that I am merely the translator of his ideas in this book.

Additionally, I must also emphasize that the book to follow is written from Ted's own point of view and in his voice.

And, of course, for anyone with more questions after reading this book, these may be posed and directly answered by Ted from Bangkok and others either on the Latest Posts page or on the Latest Questions page at the Earth Clinic website.

Bill Thompson
San Fernando
The Philippines
March 2012

* All italicized words are defined in the Resource Appendix – in the last chapter.

CHAPTER 1:

UNDERSTANDING ALKALYZING

"And we have made of ourselves living cesspools, and driven doctors to invent names for our diseases." – Plato (424-347 B.C.)

This chapter is essential reading if you want to learn what Alkalizing and Health are all about in relation to everyday life. Here you will find deeper explanations for why you need to alkalize, and the simple need for Acid/Alkali balance will be fully explained. But there is much more to learn than just balancing body pH. In this section, newer and additional essential alkalizing and health concepts will all be fully explained, including a simple group of monitoring methods using various accepted and relatively simple scientific methods and parameters, by which the user can easily monitor the ongoing state of his or her own health. This latter method and concept is a hugely important breakthrough and can be used in conjunction with alkalizing or any herbal treatments or even conventional medical treatments to discover and verify whether they are actually working or are a success. This book will, therefore, ultimately help to put you more in charge of your own health.

What is Alkalizing?

Alkalizing is a natural method of maintaining the health of the body, through supplementing with a variety of natural body-friendly alkaline nutrients, in order to promote and achieve the human body's correct healthy state through adjustment of several important body parameters. These body parameters include Conductivity, pH, ORP and Brix measurements. Through both using alkalizing techniques and monitoring these body parameters, we are able to adjust our body's poor health state back into the proper health zone with reduced body acidity, more efficient metabolism and a raised and much stronger immune system.

These monitoring methods are defined below:

Conductivity or TDS is used as an electrical urine measurement in microsiemens to determine the concentration of minerals and water in your body. TDS means Total Dissolved Solids. These minerals are all dissolved in water, so this measurement determines whether your body has the right amount of minerals in the right amount of water. A conductivity measurement that is too low tells you that you are low in body minerals, and a conductivity that is too high means that your body needs more water for better health. A healthy conductivity reading is between 4200 – 4900 microsiemens.

pH is a logarithmic measurement between 1 to 14 where 7 is neutral. Any value below 7 is acid and any value above 7 is alkaline. A pH value of 1 is the strongest acid and a pH value of 14 represents the strongest alkali. The healthy pH range is between 6.1 – 6.8.

Brix is a refractometer reading that determines the amount of sugar dissolved in a urine sample. This allows you to monitor, track and balance your own sugar levels in the blood for good health. The average healthy reading is 1.5 whereas a reading of 5 is diabetic.

ORP or Oxidation/Reduction Potential, measured in millivolts, identifies whether your body is in a potentially oxidative (cationic) state or in a potentially reductive (anionic) state. To illustrate more fully, in nature a dead or dying organism always tends to an oxidative or cationic state, whereas a healthy living body is generally in a reductive or anionic state. A healthy ORP reading is between 100 – 110 millivolts.

As you can see, alkalizing methods also have a logical and very important monitoring and tracking side involving specific scientific measurements. So these measuring tools usefully represent and define various degrees of sickness and health. These measurements and the conclusions we draw from them are all thoroughly backed by logic and scientific research and can be used as proof or as an indicator of success in the use of alkalizing or for any other healing remedy.

Some examples of how maintaining proper pH levels benefits the body are given here:

- Improves chelation and promotes removal of heavy metals from the body

- Increases the oxygenation of the body

- Reduces tissue pain by reducing acidity

- Reduces general pain by neutralizing lactic acid - a major cause of pain

- Reduces constipation caused by acidity

- Reduces diarrhea caused by excess body alkalinity

- Healthy blood pressure depends on proper nitric oxide levels, acidity destroys it

- Blood vessel constriction causes high blood pressure if the body is too acid

- Excess arterial clogging due to acidity causes strokes

- Excess acidity — below pH 6 — causes kidney dysfunctions and damage

- Sports fatigue is due to acidity build up in the body

- Recovery from strokes is dependent on achieving proper body alkalinity

- Free radicals build up occurs as acidity levels increase

- Glycation, glaucoma, and cataracts increase as body acidity increases

- Virus, fungus and other pathogen communities grow and proliferate in the body when body pH is too acid

- Pancreas function depends on bicarbonate, without which pancreatic beta cells get destroyed.

It must be stressed that the above represents only a partial list defining the benefits of alkalizing the body. Other health-giving aspects of alkalizing are further discussed in more depth in the following sections below.

The Many Benefits of Alkaline Metals and Diet

Modern medicine, especially human medicine, does not attempt to get people to control their pH within an alkaline range. This can be significant, not just in our own health, but this can also be observed in the foods we eat. For example, an excerpt from Science Daily regarding the purchasing habits of Japanese consumers at the butcher's display case:

> "...the Japanese were selecting not by color, but by what color indicated: pH, a measure of acidity or alkalinity. Darker pork has a slightly higher pH than lighter pork. A higher pH means there's less acid – acid that damages muscle proteins and causes meat to be pale and watery." – Source: Science Daily

Now just imagine what happens to your body if you don't care what happens to your pH or do not make the effort to take baking soda and citric acid to alkalize your body. Your muscles, maybe even your heart, become damaged from weakened proteins and your entire body ages much quicker. If your heart muscle breaks down, one can imagine the possibility of heart disease. Perhaps muscle aches and pains are a part of the destructive process of our muscle protein breaking down due to acid pH. pH nutrition therefore is important.

Even the pork industry now recognizes the advantages of producing pigs with alkaline pH levels to get them healthier. It therefore makes sense that to prevent our body's own proteins from breaking down that the goal of an alkaline pH doesn't only cover the pork we eat, but also alkalinity's effect on our own bodies.

Bowel Movements an Inadequate Yardstick

Bowel movements are a poor measurement of optimal health, while the body's pH balance is more important. A blood pH, if it varies only a very tiny amount with a change in blood pH of 0.5, will mean certain death. Fortunately, the kidneys act like a shock absorber excreting all our excess pH, along with the body's other poisonous byproducts.

Yet if the urinary pH is more than 8.0 (too alkaline) the bowel movements increase, resulting in diarrhea and poor digestion. If your body's pH is below 6 (too acid) this is dangerous and manifests as constipation and infection. If the pH is 5.5 then the body is stressed, but if the pH is below 5.5 this can mean possible kidney disease because the high acidity of the urine tends to digest the kidneys.

While, as you can see, the body's bowel movements are somewhat related to pH, diets vary and with them bowel behavior. Ayurveda has not yet discovered the importance of maintaining optimal pH because pH meters were not used by ancient Indians. So if you want diet guidelines that are one size fits all, monitor your pH and vary your personal diet accordingly.

The ultimate lesson here is that the human body, contrary to current medical thinking, is not always capable of maintaining perpetual internal balance or homeostasis. In our modern world of toxic, chemically processed foods the point is made that we must therefore act to continually protect our bodies from both lack of nutrients and overabundance of chemical poisons as part of helping the body in achieving correct homeostasis, in order to aid our body terrain in finally achieving sustained health.

While we humans don't agree as to what perfectly constitutes a healthy diet, we do at least all accept that high fiber diets are good for us and that proper health relies on getting the right amount of water but equally on maintaining the right pH. Bowel movements are very much related to pH, bacteria from food sources, nitrate toxicity, and optimal dietary intake more than anything else. As a result, I cannot say how many bowel movements are good for your own particular body.

What I am sure about is we don't eat enough complex carbohydrates; instead we eat too much meat and not enough fish. We should also stay away from supermarket vegetable oils. All the usual rules apply, but one added rule is to eat low energy high bulk food—which means fewer calories and a fuller stomach. The foods we eat today are generally energy dense, nutritionally lacking foods. The point being, fiber is good for you and there is really no such thing as too many healthy bowel movements; so don't count your bowel movements but count your pH, because an unhealthy bowel with low, acidic pH will be a wonderful breeding ground for dangerous pathogens.

For nearly 25 years, I have been controlling my body's pH level, mostly intuitively. And it has helped me survive colds, flu etc. because of this. Therefore, I recently decided to get myself a small electronic pH meter in order to measure both my salivary pH and urinary pH.

These units are quite revealing about your health. The ideal urinary pH and salivary pH have to be BOTH 6.5 pH, this being the minimum to achieve, but it is ideal to reach a pH of 7.0 (neutral on the acid/alkaline pH scale) if possible. Why this is so important is that this is the best pH at which your body will absorb minerals. Also, whenever salivary/urinary pH is off, this means that your body is either too acidic or too alkaline. We check our pH levels in two bodily fluids because salivary pH indicates digestive enzyme problems while urinary pH registers proper or improper mineral balance. For example, recently I had a bad pain in my leg. After testing my urinary pH, it was acidic while the saliva in my mouth was pH 6.8. This means that the body is trying to get rid of excess acidity. So I therefore decided to supplement myself with 1-2 teaspoons of sodium bicarbonate and some potassium bicarbonate. Magnesium bicarbonate is what your body needs within the cell, but this is harder to make because I would need to mix magnesium carbonate with soda water.

A simpler way is to use magnesium chloride. On the other hand, if the urinary pH is highly alkaline (or very acidic) and the salivary pH is also acidic then this means that there is a likelihood of cancer, or a fungal infection. This is a dangerous situation and reveals that your body desperately needs anionic minerals, such as magnesium, potassium, or sodium. Calcium is a tricky issue, but you need it in smaller amounts. Also it reveals the need to alkalize and to reduce protein intake.

Testing Conductivity and pH

There are other examples of what we can learn about our own health by testing the bodily fluids. I also bought a urinary conductivity meter, which measures in the unit of microsiemens as a unit of conductivity. If you were to do a urinary conductivity check, this would reveal if your urine was too conductive – which is a problem for me – because this means that I do not drink enough water. If the urinary conductivity on the other hand is below normal, which is quite common for people in the United States, it means mineral depletion or electrolyte depletion, which is common amongst athletes. Usually the average urine conductivity is between 4200-4900 microsiemens. My urinary conductivity recently went over the roof at 9500 microsiemens, which revealed that my kidneys could fail from unnecessary work since I don't drink that much water, especially during the evening hours, or this could also reveal high exposure to heavy metals, usually from faucets.

There is also a superstition that I will disprove based on my experiments with urinary conductivity. It is a commonly held belief that you should not drink water when you are eating food since you will dilute the digestive juices (lowering necessary acidity). But based on my test of this eating habit, my urinary conductivity went over the roof (over 9000 microsiemens), which means that if you do not drink while eating food, you could destroy your kidneys since the urinary mineral concentrations are far greater than nature intended and so the kidneys must work far too hard.

The reason is simple. Most foods we eat are already too high in sodium chloride (table salt) as it is, therefore these problems do not lie with digestive juices, these problems lie with you killing your kidneys! Also, my salivary pH went acid (less than pH of 6) whenever I tried not to drink water while I was eating.

Based on these tests, it seems that the most important lesson is to use urinary conductivity to measure the ideal amount of water you should drink, while your pH is used to determine whether your body is properly absorbing the required minerals from the foods we eat. Additionally, pH always seems to go off the mark before I get sick. So these meters can really be used for prevention as well. Acidic pH also reveals you are eating too much junk food, meats or snacks. These meters will therefore also tell you what to eat.

Another lesson I learned from using the pH meter is that my body is most acidic between 2:00 am to 3:00 am. This is the time when your body has its maximum toxic load. That is why it is necessary to hydrate very well before sleep and why I take some baking soda if my pH suddenly becomes acidic during the night, because this is the time when your body needs to alkalize. Also, it is probably the reason why most people die between 2 am and 3 am. When they sleep, the body's toxic load is at maximum and people don't drink enough water before they sleep or alkalize their blood before they sleep.

The other side of maintaining homeostasis – measured in terms of conductivity – is our electrolyte balance, and for us that largely means sodium chloride, or table salt. Over 80% of all macro-mineral electrolytes in blood serum consist of sodium, which is the proper balance for sodium in the body. Refined and processed salt is bad for us, however, since it adds to the acidity in our bodies. Regrettably, for nearly a century, ever since processed foods were born, this refined salt has become a staple in our diets.

Nearly concurrently, beginning fifty or so years ago, there was the scare that this high salt diet would contribute to high blood pressure and heart disease, so half of us eliminated salt and sodium from our diets. But lack of salt just as well as too much refined salt can cause major electrolyte problems for the body. This is throwing the baby out with the bathwater. Chlorides are needed for the production of hydrochloric acid in the stomach for digestion (though only in very small amounts). More critically, the sodium pump is used all over the body, in intestinal absorption and in every cell to promote mineral absorption and mineral balance. If not enough salt is taken in via our diet, then this will upset the water/mineral balance of the cells and blood, contributing to less water in the blood and blood thickening.

Rather than give up salt entirely, then, we should switch to natural sea salt, which contains a greater range of extra minerals from the sea and is more alkaline and beneficial for the body. In a person with healthy kidney, sodium then is kept in balance and excreted easily and regularly. The point here is that your body needs sodium and easily excretes any excess.

Even the healthiest table salt, however, necessarily contains chloride in its molecules, and this makes it very different from sodium bicarbonate, which offers us the needed sodium and bicarbonate without the excessive supply of chlorides. So, with a healthy kidney, there should be few problems in taking sodium bicarbonate with water for the body. The benefits for the body, as already described, are wide-ranging and numerous. The blood is alkalized, the intestines are alkalized, fat metabolism becomes more efficient, the bioavailabilty of beneficial nutrient metal salts is increased and solubility and absorption of these same are also increased so that heavy metals are more easily chelated out of the body. Since the pH is raised respiration also becomes more efficient, therefore there is more energy for the body.

Similarly, sodium and potassium citrates work to alkalize the intracellular environment, improving the cell diffusion, absorption and assimilation of essential minerals, helping to produce energy and amino acid building blocks via the Citric Acid Cycle and to help promote and maintain normal and healthy aerobic respiration in the cells.

The sodium and potassium issues are further complicated by the fact that high blood pressure is due to the presence of negative ion species such as Cl^- and $SO3^-$ (sulfites in particular). The body tries to compensate for this to get the pH back to normal with retention of positive ions (sodium, potassium, magnesium, and phosphorous) to lower the blood pressure, leading often to sodium retention. In their alkaline form sodium, potassium, magnesium and phosphorus (e.g. monopotassium phosphate, dipotassium phosphate etc.) all get retained! Unfortunately, excess phosphates in the diet lead to a rapid heartbeat, and that is what leads to high blood pressure.

To make the case more clear, if we are exposed to chlorine in the drinking water, then sulfites used as food preservatives (bisulfites, sulfites, etc.) and also something as simple as industrially made salt (which contains true chloride ions, but its pH is an unnatural pH of 5) get retained. I gave myself high blood pressure on purpose (it took more than a year eating a standard American diet) to get it to 200/100. Then I tested every one of these mineral elements, which has led to these conclusions:

1. Alkalinity is required to lower your blood pressure.

2. The effect of lower blood pressure is in the following order: potassium, magnesium, phosphate, and sodium, i.e. potassium tends to help lower blood pressure the most and sodium has the least lowering effect.

3. A state of alkalinity can mostly be achieved with the sodium since the extracellular fluids are dominated by sodium. Potassium, magnesium, and phosphate in that order (after sodium) can further increase overall alkalinity.

4. Potassium alkalinity is limited by the amount of potassium required in the body, and only after the body is sufficiently alkalized via sodium. But sodium plays a dominant part in alkalinity. Therefore, in the body, sodium and potassium must be balanced.

5. Sodium retention is also controlled by lithium, as in lithium carbonate, in smaller 1 mcg – 5 mcg dosages only and not in 250 mg dosages (the amounts used in the medical establishment to treat bipolar disorder).

6. Since chlorides are the main element driving high blood pressure, chloride compounds are excluded when fighting high blood pressure, including magnesium chloride and potassium chloride but also other species that are on the right side of the periodic table. The blood lowering effects can be derived from those elements (mostly, but not all) to the left side of the periodic table, with the exception of calcium, which has a tendency to accumulate and causes long-term (not short-term) high blood pressure.

7. Because our society has been exposed to both chlorides as well as primary and secondary acids, which leads to excess sodium — all of this leads to high blood pressure. But chlorides force the body to retain sodium in an attempt to get the body within narrow pH ranges.

8. The issue of pain is so common in human society and this is an acid problem. It is the acid in our body that leads to pain and inflammation. Cancer pain, specifically, is because of lactic acid being produced or else where there is lack of circulation, which leads to pain because that area is consequently acidic.

9. Phosphorus leads to the heart beating faster, and magnesium and potassium lead to a lower heart rate.

10. Too much sodium in the form of carbonates leads to kidney pain but, with potassium, the effect is nullified.

As you can see, I can reduce blood pressure and get it normalized my way, recognizing that the major cause of this problem is chlorides, especially the acidic forms such as common table salt (its pH is 5, not 7). Thus the question of whether the sodium in sodium bicarbonate is a threat to our health is answered in the negative.

The Benefits of Alkalizing the Body

The choice of sodium bicarbonate as the main alkalizer used in these alkalizing protocols is easily explained. First, as has already been argued, sodium is very necessary to help maintain the body's correct pH because over 80% of the body's macro-electrolytes are sodium. And as has already been stated, magnesium bicarbonate is perhaps closer to the ideal, but this nutrient is much more difficult to obtain. Sodium bicarbonate, a weak alkali or base, is also very useful for converting acids such as citric acid and ascorbic acid to their more alkaline citrate and ascorbate forms respectively. Lastly, the body needs bicarbonates for the following reasons:

- The human body needs bicarbonates as part of its homeostasis mechanism to help alkalize the body and maintain body fluids within a healthy pH zone. Contrary to much current thinking, the body is not perfect at achieving homeostasis—particularly if the body is sick with a depressed immune system.

- Despite present-day fears to the contrary, the body needs sodium because it is a major and essential constituent and electrolyte of the blood serum. Sodium is essential in powering the absorption and transfer of nutrients and minerals between the blood and corporeal cells using the sodium pump mechanism and sodium transporter networks throughout the body.

- Bicarbonates are stored and secreted by the pancreas, as they are needed in the duodenum to neutralize the hydrochloric acid from the stomach chyme at mealtimes. This is in order to allow the next phase of digestion in the duodenum, where the medium must be neutral-to-alkaline for the duodenal digestive enzymes to work properly.

- Bicarbonates are an essential aid in the energy synthesis portion of the human respiration cycle, helping in the process of swapping carbon dioxide and oxygen during respiration at the blood and cellular levels.

- Before the 1930s, baking soda or sodium bicarbonate on its own in water was widely used and recommended by doctors to cure stomach digestion problems, flu and colds and was also used as toothpaste. The dosages recommended in these times were much larger than recommended here.

Alkalizing and Digestion

As for the many opinions and fears that I've come across concerning the problems caused to the stomach by taking sodium bicarbonate, this is due to a lack of understanding on how to use baking soda properly. Of course, if you take enough baking soda or sodium bicarbonate at mealtimes then this will certainly neutralize the stomach acids and cause indigestion and stomach upset.

However, if you take baking soda in half a glass of water outside mealtimes — 1 hour after a meal or at least 30 minutes before a meal — in the correct amounts and concentrations – no harm should arise.

In fact, outside mealtimes when your stomach is empty, the sodium bicarbonate will not be neutralized by stomach hydrogen chloride (HCl) because after a meal all the leftover HCl in the stomach is either re-absorbed by that organ or is neutralized by bicarbonates secreted from the stomach lining itself (that's right, the stomach also produces sodium bicarbonate). Also, all the mucus from the lungs, throat and nose accumulates in the stomach, which further helps to protect the stomach lining against acid damage. So, if you take sodium bicarbonate outside mealtimes, it will not be neutralized and should not cause any problems whatsoever in the stomach, provided it is empty and you are not hungry.

Similarly, sodium bicarbonate can be taken in water about a half an hour or an hour or so after eating a meal – depending on the size of the meal – when all the food has completely left the stomach and moved into the duodenum for alkaline stage digestion. By taking sodium bicarbonate like this after a meal, this actually aids digestion by ensuring proper alkalization of the digestive juices, allowing proper main stage enzyme digestion in the duodenum. Sodium bicarbonate can be used in this manner if bicarbonates are lacking in the pancreatic juices.

Moreover, if you are eating a very acidic diet – for instance mixing excessive fruit juices with high amounts of proteins at mealtimes – the alkaline digestion that must occur in the duodenum may not happen because the pancreas might not have enough alkaline bicarbonates in its juices to neutralize both the stomach acids and the acidic foods eaten, in order for the main duodenal alkaline digestion to occur. In this case, problems will arise due to the constant acid diet over the longer term leading to acidic intestines and problems like IBS, colitis, candida, leaky gut and allergies. That's why, if you are eating acidic foods, then adding a little sodium bicarbonate – say 1/16 to 1/8 tsp to your drinking water at mealtimes – will help to neutralize the excess acid from the food to allow proper and balanced alkaline digestion in the duodenum to occur later. Another example is apple cider vinegar, which is considered excessively acid by some but is more palatable if some baking soda is added.

The Allopathic Viewpoint

Medical research today, for the most part, does not support or at least does not champion oral use of sodium bicarbonate or citrates as useful natural supplements for all-around health of the body. Most of the beneficial alkaline properties of these salts have been suppressed or are regarded as trivial by mainstream medical research. But before modern medicine, sodium bicarbonate was widely used orally and in much larger daily amounts than we recommend in this book.

Furthermore, alkaline salts such as sodium bicarbonate are actually widely used – and in much larger doses – by IV, injection and orally by medical professionals today. Here are some examples.

- As an oral antacid in many products.

- Via IV infusion as a flush or buffer for cancer chemotherapy.

- For women in labor suffering acidosis caused by heavy internal muscle contractions during childbirth.

- For metabolic acidosis as a serum alkalizer.

- As an alkalizing agent in prolonged cardio-pulmonary resuscitation and in the neutralization of certain intoxicants.

- As a hydration agent for radiographic contrast dyes.

- As supplementation for renal tubular acidosis in the kidneys.

- As treatment for pulmonary hypertension in newborn babies.

- As a treatment for diabetic keto-acidosis.

- As treatment for hyperkalemia (excess potassium).

Perhaps now we can more easily understand why sodium bicarbonate has so many undoubted uses in modern medicine today – since all are connected with alkalizing the body. Dr. Tullio Simoncini, an Italian oncologist, has also found that using sodium bicarbonate orally, by IV or injection can help to resolve and cure cancers. This is perhaps evidence enough of sodium bicarbonate's ability to help benefit the body in order to maintain and achieve healthy alkaline balance in the blood.

The medical view has long assumed that the human body is almost always in proper balance – because the medical establishment regards the body's ability to maintain alkaline homeostasis as having a nearly infinite capacity. Given that error, it unavoidably follows that allopathic medicine would fail to see the common and cumulative damages on our health from diets that insufficiently support the body's alkalizing needs.

Conclusions and Summary

Finally, in this chapter we have investigated the nature and reasons of how the Alkaline Metals contribute to the healthy alkaline levels in our body. Furthermore, we have described the full benefits of alkalizing in terms of the chemical and electro-chemical natures of these Alkaline Metals, which have included body pH, ORP, Conductivity and Brix measurements, to help us clarify all the reasons and to provide us with a means to actually monitor our own health state.

Put simply and generally, alkalizing the body will give the following health benefits:

- Puts the body into a much healthier pH range

- Improves malabsorption issues in the body

- Helps to remove toxins

- Helps to reduce pain in the body

- Improves digestion

- Helps to oxygenate the body

- Helps to prevent mutation abnormalities in the body's DNA

- Improves body energy

- Improves blood circulation

- Improves the electrochemistry of the body

- Improves the Redox potential of the body – making the body less oxidative

- Improves and supports the Immune System

- Creates a bad environment for pathogens

- Improves and supports body Homeostasis

In the next chapter, the particular alkalizing remedies I prefer to use myself and most strongly propose for general use will be specifically explained.

CHAPTER 2:

TED'S ALKALYZING REMEDIES

"Poison is in everything, and no thing is without poison. The dosage makes it either a poison or a remedy." — Paracelsus (1493-1591)

What should have become very clear from the last chapter is that alkalizing does not just involve or rely on adjusting your pH in order to improve your health. Alkalizing makes use of the simple alkaline metal salts to be discussed in this chapter while additionally requiring us to continually monitor the body's Conductivity, pH, ORP and Brix levels. Using these specific but simple and cheap electro-chemical monitoring methods, which are further described in the next chapter, enables you to accurately fine-tune and adjust your own individual diet and alkalizing regimen accordingly toward a healthy outcome. This is very important to understand because this enables people to take charge of their own body terrain and health.

These alkalizing methods are all-important because they also aid in detoxing the body, further acting to support and strengthen the electro-chemical nutrient gradients and transporter pathways between the cells and the blood. These alkalizing methods also help to support the Citric Acid Cycle for energy generation, which thereby works to provide more energy, more efficiently, to the cells. So the whole body benefits and you are simply healthier because of these protocols.

All the alkalizing methods below are specifically designed to alkalize both the blood and the intracellular environments (though each version may be better at targeting a specific part of the body terrain)—you must alkalize both to achieve proper levels of health. These alkalizing methods will also importantly act to bring your pH, ORP, Brix and Conductivity values to healthier levels. It must also be remembered that proper nutrient balance through diet, detoxing and removal of poisons such as heavy metals and halogens is also important and key to health recovery.

The beneficial effects of these alkalizing methods, in terms of their usefulness, are extensive and their full scope is beyond that of this book. For more details on uses and cures from these alkalizing remedies, please refer to this link on Ted's Alkalizing Formulas at the EarthClinic site.

Please also note that when sodium bicarbonate is added to the various remedies below to change the lemon/lime or ACV or citric acid form into their beneficial chemical salts in solution – or citrates and acetates respectively – this is when the mixture will fizz. In all such instances, in order to make these remedies correctly, the sodium bicarbonate or baking soda should be added until the fizzing stops.

Sodium Bicarbonate – Alkalizing the Blood

This method represents the cheapest and simplest way to alkalize the blood. All you use in this remedy is sodium bicarbonate or baking soda and water. The dosage is 1/4 to 1/2 teaspoon of sodium bicarbonate in a half glass of water normally taken 2 to 3 times a day. This remedy has a variety of uses. You can take it every day to improve health or just for maintenance. Or you can take it for a specific reason alongside other remedies. I take this remedy quite often just to keep my blood reasonably alkaline and to replenish my bicarbonate stores in the body. But you can also take this remedy a half hour after eating (no food in the stomach) to specifically alkalize acid foods that you eat and to help the duodenum to digest all the food efficiently during main stage alkaline digestion, preventing acid problems. You can also take baking soda and water 30 minutes before you eat (usually at dinner) to help reduce appetite so that you eat less.

1/4 to 1/2 tsp baking soda
4 oz water

It is also possible to take this remedy about an hour before sleep at night. This will help you to sleep and also aids the body's homeostasis or body balancing mechanisms during sleep mode by alkalizing the blood.

Sodium Bicarbonate with Lemon/Lime – Intracellular Alkalization

This is the main method for alkalizing the intracellular environment. What this remedy does is to improve the absorption of nutrients and removal of waste metabolites to and from the cells respectively. Lemons and limes also contain citric and ascorbic acids – which are first converted to their post-digested forms in the remedy – to citrates and ascorbates – by simply adding sodium bicarbonate to these juices. Thus you can easily take this remedy between meals without wasting your own body's bicarbonates through digestion. As well, lemons and limes have healthy amounts of macro-minerals like magnesium and potassium as well as important micro-minerals, all of which are beneficial to bodily and cellular processes.

> 1 lemon or lime
> 1/4 to 1/2 tsp baking soda
> 4 oz water

The dosage is 1 lemon or 1 lime (approximately two tablespoons of juice) to be squeezed and the juice added to half a glass of water, and then 1/4 to 1/2 teaspoon of baking soda is added until the fizzing stops. Taken twice a day on an empty stomach.

A variation of this remedy exists for people with sodium issues: one whole freshly squeezed lemon (or lime) and keep adding the bicarbonate until the fizz stops. In this case, the bicarbonate should be made of 50/50, sodium bicarbonate and potassium bicarbonate. Sodium must always be there to achieve somewhat of a sodium/potassium balance. Take this twice a day, once in the morning and once in the evening, on an empty stomach. This is done to avoid diarrhea problems, which may result if taken along with food.

Organic Apple Cider Vinegar and Sodium Bicarbonate

This is also alkalizing and can be used extensively and specifically for a whole host of other problems like GERD, fibromyalgia (with magnesium), liver problems and lack of energy. The dosage is 2 tablespoons of apple cider vinegar (ACV) in half a glass of water with 1/4 to 1/2 teaspoon of baking soda. Add the baking soda until the fizzing stops. This remedy is taken twice a day on an empty stomach.

> 2 Tbsp apple cider vinegar
> 1/4 to 1/2 tsp baking soda
> 4 oz water

Many people take raw and undiluted organic ACV, which is an older way, but this will have certain effects that are not beneficial to the body. ACV is quite acidic and tends to burn the oesophagus and also creates holes or cavities in teeth when constantly taken raw this way. When the raw ACV – which contains acetic and malic acids – reaches the duodenum it is converted into their alkaline salts – malates and acetates – due to the bicarbonates in the pancreatic juices. By adding the sodium bicarbonate before you take ACV, you are taking the safer alkaline salts form or the post-digested form of ACV and there will be no unpleasant problems with the teeth or oesophagus. As well, you will not be using up your important body bicarbonates from the pancreatic juices, as you would with raw ACV, to convert the ACV to its salt form in the duodenum. So taking ACV with sodium bicarbonate actually also helps to conserve your own body's bicarbonates, which are important for alkalizing the body.

Citric Acid with Sodium Bicarbonate and Potassium Bicarbonate

This is another variation to accommodate excess sodium or potassium shortage issues and is similar to the lemon/lime protocol. The dosage is 1/4 teaspoon citric acid crystals with 1/8 teaspoon sodium bicarbonate and 1/16 teaspoon potassium bicarbonate. This is normally taken twice a day on an empty stomach.

1/8 tsp sodium bicarbonate
1/16 tsp potassium bicarbonate
¼ tsp Citric Acid Crystals
4 oz water

The Carbicarb Remedy

This remedy consists of taking 1/2 teaspoon of sodium bicarbonate, 1/4 teaspoon sodium carbonate and 1/8 teaspoon of potassium carbonate in a half glass of water. This remedy is particularly useful for those who have lack of potassium or excess sodium issues.

1/2 tsp sodium bicarbonate
1/4 tsp sodium carbonate
1/8 tsp potassium carbonate
4 oz water

This remedy is more alkaline and can also penetrate the blood/bone and blood/brain barriers to specifically help alkalize these regions. For instance insomnia or apnea issues can be caused by acidic brain fluids, and this remedy will help to alkalize the brain itself, which tends to relax the brain. This can be taken outside mealtimes for more extensive alkalization of the body's peripherals and/or taken an hour or so before sleep for insomnia or apnea problems.

Alkalizing – More Proof of Safety

Further proof of safety with respect to these alkalizing ingredients is given in the Resource Appendix section at the end of the book. Here the Material Safety Data Sheets (MSDS) – which are the bible for defining the toxicity and handling of any chemical – for all the chemicals used in these alkalizing remedies are compared to the toxicity of common table salt.

CHAPTER 3:
MONITORING AND
TRACKING YOUR OWN
HEALTH

"It's supposed to be a secret, but I'll tell you anyway. We doctors do nothing. We only help and encourage the doctor within." – Albert Schweitzer, M.D.

This section further explains the health benefits to be had in making regular use of the previously noted four ways to track your own health by using ORP, Conductivity, pH and Brix meter readings. These monitoring and tracking methods essentially reveal your own health condition in terms of an acid/alkaline body, body mineral/water balance, body oxidation/reduction state and glucose levels.

How to Track Your Own Health

In my own personal opinion, I think Conductivity is the most important reading since it monitors the level of urine conductivity. This is important on two counts. First, if the conductivity is too high, it shows that you don't drink enough water or that your urine contains high levels of heavy metals. Second, if conductivity is too low then you might have a mineral imbalance or electrolyte depletion. On the other hand, your body may not properly be hydrated and you could be destroying your kidneys from overwork if the conductivity is too high. The second most important meter is the pH meter, which of course monitors your salivary pH (digestive system) and urinary pH (mineral balance) by keeping your pH ideally at 6.4 (the allowable range is pH 6.1-6.8). At this range all major minerals (potassium, magnesium, calcium, molybdenum, etc.) are most readily absorbed by the body. If your pH is acidic, you will suffer from colds, bacterial infections, fungi, antibiotic toxicity etc. But if your body is too alkaline then digestion will become inefficient and there will be too much ammonia in the blood from excessive protein breakdown. This leads to neurotoxicity as exemplified by problems such as ADHD. Any values above or below optimum will indicate mineral and electrolyte imbalance.

The ORP meter is a popular meter in the alternative health field, which measures whether your body is in a reducing or oxidizing state. While this is a complicated measurement, what I do know is that your body's ORP should be lower than that of water.

What this means is that if your urinary ORP measurement is more positive than -50 millivolts then you are aging rapidly. The antioxidants are lacking. This means that you are electron deficient and that your body's anionic/cationic ratios are badly balanced, so you need to take anionic mineral supplements such as magnesium, potassium, sodium, and most importantly vitamin C! You also need to drink dechlorinated, defluorinated water.

However, if your ORP exceeds minus 110 millivolts (too negative) for your urinary ORP, it might mean that you are eating too many anionic foods, which is rare, or too much vitamin C. The exception is me because I myself am overdoing it because of the fear of cationic (oxidative) foods, medicines etc. But 90% of our processed foods and medicines are cationic and not very health promoting, as this is very oxidative for the body.

In general, I would conclude that ORP looks at how fast your body is aging or degrading and this depends on how close it is to the positive ORP range. When your body is oxidizing it also means that you might have heavy metal toxicity with maybe a positive ORP as well. This means there are a lot of free metal radicals accumulating in your body and you may need EDTA therapy to remove the heavy metals out of your body. Otherwise, a long length of time with a near-positive ORP may mean an impending heart attack. Here, oral EDTA might help. The product I use is disodium EDTA. Of course, chlorinated and fluoridated water causes high positive ORP readings also and you may have to remove this from your food supply.

The fourth meter is the Refractometer or Brix, which checks your sugar level. The optimum urinary Brix is about 1.5.

As you can guess these are all pretty straightforward devices. They will help tell you when, what, and how much you should eat and drink. They tell you what is causing your health problems from what kind of foods your body is not accepting. It will also tell you whether all those supplements you are taking are any good and indicate what food is good for you and what foods are bad for you. These devices will also tell you that you are getting sick even before you are sick. In other words, they tell you a lot!

Because of my recent experiments with bean sprouts, I find it necessary to ALWAYS add hydrogen peroxide to the water I drink. It helps to alternate days with a dechlorinator (only sodium thiosulfate please!) and a fluoride inhibitor (sodium tetraborate (borax) or sodium perborate). A possible fluoride remover is magnesium oxide (but you must leave it in water for 48 hours) which is too long for me, so borax would be better.

Now the above information is not all-inclusive. If your urine has an ammonia smell, it means your body needs potassium bicarbonate supplements. Most diets are potassium deficient. There is also a possibility that you are hydrochloric acid deficient. Another way to reduce the ammonia smell of urine is to take ascorbic acid or vitamin C in acid form (ascorbic acid) with glutamine.

Adjusting Your pH Balance

From experimenting on myself and monitoring all these indicators, I have found that the best way to control pH at the optimal range is to use potassium bicarbonate and sodium bicarbonate. These are two very practical ways to get your acidic pH urine/saliva up to the optimum, because the fact is that our diets are usually acidic. This is a problem, because acids burn out our cells and cause accelerated aging. Fortunately, bicarbonate is slightly alkaline and provides the bicarbonate in the diet needed by the body. The best time to take it is whenever your pH is most acidic, which is ordinarily during the night. It is best used when pH is around 5.6-5.9 (urinary). However if the pH is below that then somewhat stronger akalinity is needed. In which case, I turn to a potassium carbonate, potassium bicarbonate and sodium bicarbonate mixture. So if you take these, then both your salivary and urinary pH optimum readings should be closely aligned. The usual dosage for me is 1/2 teaspoon of potassium bicarbonate, 1/2 - 1 teaspoon of sodium bicarbonate. But if my pH is very acid, I add 1/8 teaspoon of potassium carbonate as well.

Magnesium is also very important as a natural alkalizing agent, but I take it in the form of magnesium chloride instead of the more complicated magnesium bicarbonate. The reason I haven't mentioned anything about magnesium bicarbonate is the difficulty of making it. This method consists of using one tablespoon of magnesium carbonate to be dissolved in a closed bottle of soda water (you use one of those 1.5 to 2 liter bottles of soda). Once the cloudy solution is cleared you are done. If it remains cloudy you may need to add more soda water.

In rare instances of those people whose pH readings are alkaline (which means that their pH goes over 7), then it means your digestion is not working. In this case you need to make your body more acidic. The best way, at least for me, is to take vitamin C or sodium acetate (which is vinegar and baking soda mixed together), which is slightly acidic. On the other hand, you can just take vinegar or apple cider vinegar raw if you like.

All of these methods of stabilizing your pH are simply a quick fix; however, for in the long run the best way is to eat more alkali forming foods if you are acidic and eat more acid forming foods if you are alkaline.

The easy way to remember what foods are acid forming or alkali forming is simple: acid forming foods are protein foods (chicken, pork, beef, eggs etc.) and starches, while alkali forming are vegetarian foods (nuts, vegetables, and fruits).

The reason why we get cancer, viruses etc. usually has very much to do with eating too much of acid forming foods. Additionally, when we eat acid forming foods we also get high nitrates, ammonia wastes, etc. and these are very hard for our body to get rid of, as they cause constipation. On the flip side, if we eat too many alkali forming foods we get groggy, tired and weak. So moderation is best.

For those people who measure pH you will find that you will constantly (almost everyday) have to alkalize your body because we have obviously a very bad diet, even for health-conscious people, as most foods are acidic and hard to avoid but if you have access to vegetarian diets then that is a great help.

For those people who measure conductivity and find it too high, you will find that you have to take water a lot more often (especially in the night), particularly if you are taking supplements or if the local water supply has heavy metals. For most people, I would imagine that their conductivity will be low, in which case they will have to take mineral supplements or perhaps fulvic acid as well as electrolyte minerals.

It is a bitter learning experience, as these meters will reveal, because we simply don't take care of our bodies as well as we take care of our shiny new cars or the clothes we wear.

Measuring Your Own State of Health

Since these meters vary so widely in method of use, only the proper in-health ranges per meter will be defined below. For actual examples of meter usage, please refer to the Resource Appendix, which is the last chapter in the book.

The ORP Meter

This involves measuring the Oxidation/Reduction Potential or Redox Potential of your urine. A healthy body will have an ORP of below (more negative than) -100 millivolts (minus 100 millivolts). A more positive reading of -50 millivolts indicates poor health and a reading of less than or more positive than -15 millivolts indicates the possibility of a more serious ailment like cancer or heart disease in the body. I once measured the ORP of a cancer patient and his ORP was -20 millivolts. Obviously to fix that, I added vitamin C and N acetyl cysteine, two substances that have strong negative ORP.

Healthy ORP range: -70 to -100 millivolts.

If you measured the ORP of the Lemon and Lime or ACV with baking soda drinks, they would be in the very healthy -200 millivolt range. So if your ORP is too positive, you can alkalize back to health using these remedies over a period of time.

The Conductivity Meter

Conductivity measures both the mineral content and water content of the blood and body. This measurement is also taken on your urine. If the conductivity is too high, then you are probably lacking water in your diet, but if your conductivity measurement is too low then you are lacking proper mineral balance in your diet.

The correct healthy range is between 4200 – 4900 microsiemens.

If you lack minerals, then take a mineral supplement like fulvic/humic acid drops with macro-mineral supplements everyday until you are in the healthy range. And if you lack water – that's easy – drink more water (two glasses) at mealtimes.

The pH Meter

pH measures the acid/alkaline state of your body. Readings are taken on both your urine and saliva. Both should be in the average pH 6.4 range.

The pH range for good health is a pH of 6.1 to 6.8.

Generally, people's diets are too acidic, so taking the alkalizing remedies defined in this book will help to bring the body's pH back into the healthy alkaline range. If your urine is too acidic, take sodium bicarbonate on its own with water to alleviate this by alkalizing the blood. If your saliva is too acidic, then alkalize the intracellular environment by taking the Lemon/Lime or ACV and baking soda and water remedies two times a day until you are in the correct pH health range.

The Brix Meter or Refractometer

The Brix meter is a simple meter used to measure the glucose or sugar content of a solution by light refraction. It is often used in agriculture for things like beer in brewing and grapes in wine-making. For our purposes, the urine sugar content is normally measured.

The optimum health reading (for low body sugar) is 1.5. A Brix reading of 5 indicates that you are diabetic.

This is a way of monitoring your sugar levels so that through a proper diet you can keep them down to safer, healthier levels. From research, it is well known that large daily amounts of any sugar in the diet will drag the immune system down or turn off the immune system within 2 hours of sugar consumption. In a 2005 large-scale cancer research experiment involving over one million South Korean participants, including over 20,000 people with different cancers, it was found that those with sugar levels in the blood below 90 mgs/dL (or below 90 mgs per 100 cc) were able to survive their cancer (representing only 3% of research participants). However, it was also found that in 97% of the research participants whose sugar levels were greater than 90 mgs/dL (Brix equivalent reading is 1.5), the cancer was most likely to metastasize, spread and grow unhindered until the patient's death despite conventional treatments. Keeping glucose and fructose sugar levels down in your diet is therefore very beneficial for health. But you will also need lysine (an amino acid) to drive up the white blood cells, because these white blood cells eat cancer.

CHAPTER 4:

TED'S HEALTH DEFENCE DIET

"The doctor of the future will no longer treat the human frame with drugs, but rather will cure and prevent disease with nutrition." -- Thomas Edison

A Very Short History of the Human Diet

The modern Western Diet is effectively 90% acid-forming foods. Before 1900, and before processed foods were all the rage, there was a big difference in diet. At this time, the main fats used in diets in the West were usually lard, tallow (beef fat), and butter. Similarly in the tropical countries and in the Pacific Rim region, the main fats eaten were palm oil, coconut oil and clarified butter (ghee)— all saturated fats. In Alaska and Northern Canada, in older times, the Eskimos ate nothing but pure whale blubber, a mammalian saturated fat—and they hardly ever got heart disease or cancer as a common illness.

People might reel from these facts but, strangely, when compared to today's horrific medical statistics on disease and illness, there were far fewer numbers of people actually suffering from degenerative diseases like cancer, heart disease, high blood pressure, diabetes, Alzheimer's, CFS, obesity, heart disease and other auto-immune diseases before the 1900s than occurs today in our own modern world. Many vaccines actually trigger autoimmune diseases—that's why it occurs in developed countries. And here's something else to consider. Since the 1960s we have all been brainwashed to believe that chemically processed vegetable oils (which are mostly hydrogenated oils and trans fatty acid) are indeed good for us. But if this were the case, and everyone is cooking and eating with processed vegetable oils now (for the last 40 or so years), how come the statistical numbers for people with cancer, heart disease, diabetes etc. are still surging upwards? Surely, all these horrible medical stats should be going down shouldn't they?

Before 1900 and the worldwide introduction of heavily processed foods, there were very few refrigerators around to help preserve food. So what did people use as preservatives? People would used vinegar and herbs to pickle and preserve vegetables – like Korean kimchi – and made fruit jams and conserves whenever vegetables and fruits were seasonally available. Drying and salting was also another major method used to preserve both fish and meats throughout the world. People ate a lot more salted meats and fish – and therefore more salt than they do today – only they didn't use refined salt in those days, they simply used sea salt or rock salt – far healthier for the body because these salt forms contain a host of other beneficial minerals for our bodies. Refined salt contains nothing but NaCl—sodium chloride. In the Philippines and other countries, dried, salted fish is still a huge part of their diet. Other countries also used spices like cumin, turmeric, chili, garlic and cloves, which were all used to make beef jerky and which, when dried, preserved meats for a very long time because of the antibiotic effect of the spices. In old India, the whole point of the curry dish was not only that the spices made it taste so great, but that the spices actually helped to preserve the curry leftovers safely for many days, even weeks, in the tropical heat. If you check your freezer Food Rules and check how long you can preserve lamb curry, beef curry or chicken curry in the freezer, it's a heck of a lot longer than is allowed for ordinary raw, roasted, fried or stewed meats without these particular spices.

Old Food Cycle (pre 1850)

In conclusion, we can say that the pre-1900 American diet contained food that was more or less grown or raised on healthy, organic soils, without NPK chemical fertilizers, which always tend to acidify the soil, preventing essential macro and micro-mineral absorption by the plants. The food was therefore much more organic and alkaline in older times. There were also a lot more minerals in vegetables. Today it is known that U.S. soils are typically deficient in at least 10 major minerals. The edible oils used back then were mainly saturated fats and there was a much higher intake of natural sea or rock salt in the diet. Also, the main grains that were eaten at this time in the U.S. were mainly oats and millet (no gluten) and not wheat. Add to this that only natural organic fertilizers were used – no pesticides or fungicides – therefore their water-tables were unpolluted and naturally preserved. There was no chemical sewage transformed into drinking water – so no dangerous additives like chlorine, fluorine, pesticides or fungicides in their drinking water.

To rapidly summarize, the older pre-1900 diets really consisted of natural foods with no chemical food processing, no commercially canned foods (bisphenol A), no fungicides, no pesticides, no additives, no preservatives, no food colorings, no homogenization, no pasteurization, no irradiation, no margarine, no excessive food fortification with calcium, no excess refined sugar, no aspartame, no MSG, no synthetic vitamins, no GMO foods, no disguised E factors, no steroids, drugs or antibiotics in animal foods, no plastics used in the food industry, no fluorine or chlorine in the water supply, no brominated bread, no battery raised chickens, no feeding farm animals with unnatural foods, no medical drugs industry, no Codex Alimentarius, no RDA recommendations and no FDA.

Sick Soils = Sick Plants = Sick Animals = Sick Humans.

Modern Food Cycle

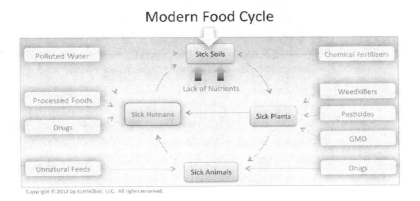

Ted's Health Defence Diet

The following diet is a nutrition guide but is not really meant as a diet at all. A diet suggests that, one day, you will come off the diet. Therefore this diet is really a Way of Eating for Life. So it really should be more specifically regarded as a defensive way of eating that both helps to protect and alkalize your body. This diet can also be easily used with ordinary Western diets or even with organic, vegetarian or vegan diets—the same guidelines apply. This diet is also recommended for problems like cancer, acid body, candida etc. on Earth Clinic. We offer it here because it is a very useful complement to Ted's Alkalizing Remedies, since this way of eating helps to alkalize, detox and to protect your body from the effects of chemically processed foods.

All the same, this diet is only meant as a set of guidelines to educate. It is up to the reader how he or she interprets and applies it. However, if you are ill with a particularly serious illness like cancer or even candida, then the full diet will be necessary and must be fully applied.

Here is the Health Defence Diet:

1. **NO SUGAR.** Cancers, viruses and all pathogens feed off sugar, which promotes their rapid growth and spread. When too much sugar is eaten constantly everyday, this habit also works to greatly lower the immune system's capability to fight disease. In particular, cancers grow in the presence of the fructose found in fruits, and to survive they need glucose.

2. **Moderate or reduced carbohydrate intake.** The Western diet is effectively an energy dense but nutrient deficient diet in terms of minerals and vitamins. Therefore for sugar-loving diseases like cancer and candida, carbohydrates are banned because they so easily convert to sugar in the body. If you can, eat carbohydrates that have a low glycemic index, which are digested and absorbed slowly in the body and which do not cause high sugar spikes in the body. These sugar spikes tend to bring down the immune system and feed the invading pathogens as well. Also beware that the Glycemic Index doesn't measure the type of sugar so is not a perfect measure or guide to go by.

2. **No junk food allowed.** Junk food contains way too much refined salt, MSG, vegetable oils and other additives. All bad.

3. **No vegetable oils in the diet.** Vegetable oils oxidize fairly quickly on the shelf from sunlight and very rapidly at high heat because they are polyunsaturated (weak chemical bonds) fats. Most RBD vegetable oils nowadays

are also made from an unnatural chemical process. As far back as 1962, Dr. Denham Harman, a Nobel Prize winner who discovered the anti-oxidant nature of vitamins, proved in his famous experiments in feeding mice vegetable oils with their food, that chemically processed vegetable oils or polyunsaturated oils significantly contribute to causing cancer. So, better to use a saturated fat like virgin coconut oil (VCO) or even grass-fed lard for cooking—saturated fats are more stable oils that do not oxidize easily and are also good for you.

Many vegetarian websites quote The Okinawan Diet as their reason for a vegetables-only eating regimen being best for you, which is inaccurate. If you read the book, The Okinawan Diet – which carefully defines this diet through the writers' research – the Okinawans generally used pork offal and pork fat in all their healthy cooking – and, in their pre-WW2 diet they never used whole grain bread, olive oil, soy milk, apples, or yogurt. When I had systemic candida and started taking coconut oil, my bad constipation and bloating issues disappeared in about two weeks and my toilet habits became regular again. VCO is very healthy for your body and intestines. I only ever cook with VCO now, and it has actually helped me to lose weight.

Since the 1960s, baby-foods have been using only coconut oil for their cooked products, and those in the hospital with intestinal trauma are usually fed with food cooked in coconut oil as well. This is because VCO helps to protect the intestines and the body while also being anti-bacterial, anti-viral and anti-fungal.

4. **No soda pop.** Apart from containing sugar, high fructose corn syrup (HFCS), fructose and aspartame, sweet soda drinks also contain carbonic and phosphoric acids as well as halogens like fluorides in their mix – all

of which only work to acidify your body. Furthermore, HFCS often contains mercury and poisonous chemicals like glutaraldehyde – which is normally used as a poisonous industrial cleaner.

5. **No artificial sweeteners—no aspartame, sucralose or saccharine.** Aspartame is acidifying. It is also an excitotoxin that helps to destroy your central nervous system. In our bodies, aspartame metabolizes into formaldehyde and methanol, which is also a poison. (In the old days people used stills to make their own illicit distilled alcoholic beverages and if they were not careful in their process methanol would form. This wood alcohol or methanol is poisonous and as little as 10 ml would be enough to cause permanent blindness.) Sucralose is a chlorinated hydrocarbon that, in tests, causes a shrunken thymus, enlarged kidneys, abortion and low fetal weights, as these areas are all sensitive to chlorine compounds in hydrocarbon forms. Saccharine, even a moderate dose, can increase the incidence of tumors in people with cancer.

6. **Eat chicken, fish and meats in small amounts.** Proteins – meats – eaten in excessive quantities are acidifying as we get older, since our body has difficulty digesting them. Proteins should preferably be partially cooked to ease the breaking down of proteins.

7. **No baked goods like bread, cakes, pastries, etc.** In the '70s the FDA, in their wisdom, allowed the use of bromide and bromates in bread-making instead of iodine. Bromine weakens the immune system and encourages an acid body state. Wheat also contains gluten and alloxan, a poison that can help to destroy the pancreas and causes diabetes over time.

8. **Add coriander/cilantro and green tea to your rou-**

tine. In your diet, include a handful of raw, chopped coriander leaf (also called cilantro) in a salad three times a week and drink green tea 2-3 times a day. Maintaining this regimen for a month will successfully remove most heavy metals from your body.

9. **No canned products in the diet.** Bisphenol A – or BPA – is a component in the plastic that lines canned goods, and is very bad for you. It acts as a pseudo-estrogen – a female hormone – and upsets hormone balance, therefore weakening the immune system.

10. **No calcium, which means no dairy products.** No milk, no cheese, no yoghurt etc. Avoid all calcium fortified foods. Excess calcium encourages acidity throughout the body and particularly in the tissue cells where it tends to cause myalgia pain. In 1970, the recommended calcium to magnesium ratio was 4:1. Then it became 2:1 in the 1990s. I'm guessing that, probably in another 10 years, these same RDA experts will recommend a calcium to magnesium ratio of 1:1. I recommend taking no calcium supplementation in your diet because Western foods are all over-fortified with calcium now. Calcium causes acidity inside the cells when taken in excess and when magnesium is lacking in the diet. Magnesium regulates calcium in the body.

11. **No Fruits.** In general most fruits contain citric acid and sugar – especially the citrus fruits. In a healthy body that can cope with the acid and sugars from fruits it is fine to eat fruits in moderation. But if you are ill with an acid-loving and sugar-loving disease like cancer then any acidic or sugary food like fruits will actually promote its spread because eating fruits uses up your alkaline body bicarbonates during digestion. This further weakens the immune system, increases blood acidity and helps diseases like cancer to dominate the body. You can eat fruit

extracts that don't contain fructose, such as red wine extract, grapeseed extract etc.

12. **No Monosodium Glutamate (MSG).** MSG is disallowed for the same reasons as aspartame. The antidote to MSG is taurine amino acid, which is mainly found in fish.

13. **Avoid GMO foods.** The most common GMO food is actually wheat. But there is also soy GMO. All soy products made from a chemical process – including soy sauce, tofu etc. – should be avoided. But any soy products made from a natural and organic fermentation process are allowed. If you buy soya products like soya milk, make sure it is organic and contains soya flour. But if it contains soya protein then it has been made from a chemical process and also might be GMO (especially in the US).

14. **Avoid distilled water and tap water.** Distilled water is "dead water"—it completely lacks the important body minerals that natural spring-water contains. If you drink distilled water, this will actually act to pull important minerals out of your body during digestion. Tap water nowadays – due to water shortages – is now recycled and chemically processed from sewage (especially in cities) and stored in reservoirs that are fed from water tables polluted with agricultural fertilizers and pesticides, so goodness knows what evil goodies tap water contains. Enough said I think. Drink fresh mineral or spring water or create your own mineral water instead. You should always drink 1 – 2 glasses of water at mealtimes. This helps digestion and will improve your urine conductivity reading, provided your body minerals are in balance.

15. **Use sea salt rather than refined table salt.** Use sea salt for all your cooking and eating needs. Sea salt

contains many beneficial natural minerals, is alkaline, and also aids nutrient absorption and acts like a protective antibiotic in the body, which helps to protect the intestines and liver. Sea salt is also far more alkaline than refined table salt, which is normally acidic.

16. **Try to avoid all (chemically) processed food.** Try to eat foods that are made from natural processes without excess heating or use of chemicals. Read food labels carefully before you buy.

17. **Eat your big meals early.** Whenever you eat your meals, it is always best to eat bigger meals at breakfast and lunch. Your evening dinner should be eaten early at about 5:00 pm because shortly after this time, your body goes into another mode. This mode slows down digestion, making it inefficient, which actually impairs digestion, such that large amounts of food can end up sitting and stagnating in your intestines for anything up to 12 hours. This results in acidity, pathogen growth and poisons being absorbed into the body from the intestines. Better as a habit to eat a much smaller quantity of food at dinner to ensure healthy and complete digestion of food before sleep.

18. **Enjoy your meals!** When you eat food, don't always rush and over-stuff yourself, as this can lead to poor, inefficient digestion and acid intestines. There is always a lag from when you feel hungry to when your hunger is satisfied, but if you eat too fast you will eat more than your body needs, and this is not good for you. Eat your food slower, chew food thoroughly, and drink plenty of water at mealtimes for proper digestion. The Chinese – and Okinawans – normally eat until they feel 70% full, then they stop. This is a good, simple dietary practice.

Facts, Advice and Feedback

The final point I would like to make is to convince the reader that doctors are not in charge of your health—you are!! And this is simply a matter of self-education and choice. That's why the alkalizing methods in this book are so unique and important. This approach gives you all the necessary means and the tools to bring your own body terrain back to health using these alkalizing and healing protocols, using health monitoring methods and adopting the Health Defence Diet guidelines. This makes it a more complete set of explained protocols. And this really does put you back in charge because it makes you the ultimate expert on your own body and your own health.

Lastly, if there are any questions arising from this book, then the reader also has the option of asking his or her particular questions directly by posting on the Latest Posts or on Latest Questions pages at the EarthClinic website. Here, Ted from Bangkok or others will endeavour to answer your questions on Alkalizing for free. Also please have a look at the Resource Appendix, the last chapter in this book, which presents many articles and reference links to supportive research as to why and how we all need to alkalize.

Finally, any feedback on EarthClinic from the reader would be honestly and gratefully appreciated because this will help to further prove and improve the efficacy of these alkalizing remedies and will, ultimately, work to convince other sick people to take charge of their own health via these useful testimonials and ultimately help them to improve their own lives.

"Natural forces within us are the true healers of disease."
Hippocrates 460 BC – 370 BC

RESOURCE APPENDIX

Definitions

Acid
A chemical substance (typically, a corrosive or sour-tasting liquid) that neutralizes alkalis, dissolves some metals, and turns litmus paper red.

Alkali
Water-soluble strong base. Alkalis feel soapy to the touch, have a pH above 7.0, and turn litmus paper blue.

Conductivity
The degree to which a specified material conducts electricity, calculated as the ratio of the current density in the material to the electric field that causes the flow of current. It is the reciprocal of the resistivity. In terms of body urine measurements, it is a measure of Total Dissolved Solids (TDS) of the solution, which represents the body mineral to water ratio.

Homeostasis
The tendency of the body to move towards a normal, optimal and healthy physiological state by automatic self-adjustment of its own internal metabolic processes.

Monomorphism
Theory that pathogens and microbes only ever have one form and one role and do not change.

ORP
This is a measure of the tendency of a chemical species to acquire electrons or to donate electrons and thereby be reduced or oxidized respectively. When used as a urine measurement, this shows whether your body is in an oxidative or reductive state and is also a measure of body degeneration or aging caused by cumulative free-radical damage.

pH
A figure expressing the acidity or alkalinity of a solution on a logarithmic scale on which 7 is neutral, values lower than 7 are more acid, and higher values are more alkaline.

Pleomorphism
Theory that pathogens and microbes can change form according to the changing state of their host environment.

RBD
Refined, Bleached and Deodorized when applied to the manufacture of edible oils and foods when this involves industrial chemical processes.

TDS
Total Dissolved Solids, an aspect of conductivity.

Advice on the Sourcing of Chemical Nutrients

Sodium Bicarbonate: Found at pharmacies and at the supermarket – in the washing and cleaning section – and it also can be bought from internet vendors.

Potassium Bicarbonate: Found at pharmacies and on the internet.

Sodium Carbonate: Can be bought at pharmacies and bought from internet vendors.
Potassium Carbonate: May be bought at pharmacies and bought from internet vendors.

Organic Apple Cider Vinegar (ACV): Purchased at supermarkets, health shops, supermarkets and internet vendors.

Citric Acid: Obtained from supermarkets in the cooking/baking section and also can be purchased from pharmacies or internet vendors.

For further helpful information on sourcing and brands, users of these alkalizing protocols should also go to the Where to Buy section (http://www.earthclinic.com/CURES/where_to_buy.html) for the various different countries and regions at EarthClinic.com for further information on sourcing nutrients in their own particular areas.

Reference Resources

Using ORP, pH, Conductivity (TDS) and Brix Meters

How to Use an ORP Meter
http://ezinearticles.com/?How-To-Use-An-ORP-Meter&id=5811649

How to Use pH Meters
http://www.ehow.com/how_4781811_use-ph-meter.html

How to Use Conductivity Meters
http://www.reefkeeping.com/issues/2004-04/rhf/feature/

How to Use a Brix Refractometer
http://www.grapestompers.com/refractometer_use.asp

Toxicity of Alkalizing Ingredients
Below are links to Material Safety Data Sheets (MSDS), the bible
for toxicity definition and substance handling, for the various main
natural chemical bases and salts used in Ted's Alkalizing Remedies.
Table salt toxicity is used as the baseline comparison.

MSDS for Salt
http://msds.chem.ox.ac.uk/SO/sodium_chloride.html

MSDS for Sodium Bicarbonate
http://msds.chem.ox.ac.uk/SO/sodium_bicarbonate.html

MSDS for Potassium Bicarbonate
http://msds.chem.ox.ac.uk/PO/potassium_bicarbonate.html

MSDS for Sodium Carbonate
http://msds.chem.ox.ac.uk/SO/sodium_carbonate_monohydrate.html

MSDS for Potassium Carbonate
http://msds.chem.ox.ac.uk/PO/potassium_carbonate_anhydrous.html

MSDS Citric Acid
http://msds.chem.ox.ac.uk/CI/citric_acid_anhydrous.html

MSDS Sodium Citrate
http://msds.chem.ox.ac.uk/SO/sodium_citrate_monobasic.html

MSDS Tripotassium Citrate
http://msds.chem.ox.ac.uk/PO/potassium_citrate_monohydrate.html

Earth Clinic Links to Ted's Alkalizing Protocols

Ted's Alkalizing Remedies
http://www.earthclinic.com/Remedies/alkalizing_formulas.html

Ted's Q & A Page on Alkalizing
http://www.earthclinic.com/Remedies/alkalizing_formulas_questions.html

Bechamp's Terrain Theory vs. Pasteur's Germ Theory

Terrain vs Germ Theory
http://www.alternativewholistichealth.com/your_terrain.php

Health Advantage
http://thehealthadvantage.com/biologicalterrain.html

Research and Articles on Alkalizing

D. Minich et al, *Acid-Alkaline Balance: Role in Chronic Disease and Detox.*
Functional Research Medical Center, Gig Harbour.
http://www.isisboston.com/assets/PDF-Files/Compilation-of-Research-Studies-1.pdf

J Charles et al, *Metabolic Acidosis*. Clinical Review Article.
http://www.turner-white.com/memberfile.php?PubCode=hp_
mar05_acid.pdf

R C Morris et al, *The Relationship and Interaction between Sodium and
Potassium*. Dept Medicine, UCLA.
http://www.jacn.org/content/25/suppl_3/262S.full.pdf

M H Rosner, *Metabolic Acidosis in Patients with Gastro-Intestinal Disorders:
Metabolic and Clinical Consequences*.
http://www.medicine.virginia.edu/clinical/departments/medicine/
divisions/digestive-health/nutrition-support-team/nutrition-articles/
RosnerArticle.pdf

M Sircus, *Mighty Mallet of Baking Soda*. Article. IMVA.
http://sodiumbicarbonate.imva.info/index.php/administration-
methods/mighty-mallet-of-baking-soda/

How Human Digestion Works. Biology Innovations.
http://www.biology-innovation.co.uk/pages/human-biology/the-
digestive-system/

Gastric Acid: Neutralization. Wikipedia.
http://en.wikipedia.org/wiki/Gastric_acid#Neutralization

M Sircus, *Sodium Bicarbonate Oral Dosages*. IMVA Article.
http://www.imva.info/news/oral-dosages-of-bicarbonate.html

M Sircus, *Sodium Bicarbonate Treatment for Swine Flu* (1924). IMVA
Article.
http://sodiumbicarbonate.imva.info/index.php/administration-
methods/arm-hammer-soda-company/

Importance of Bicarbonates and Citrates to Human Health. Magnesium
Online Library.
http://www.mgwater.com/bicarb.shtml

The Importance of Bicarbonates in Human Respiration. Tutor Vista w/s.
http://www.tutorvista.com/content/biology/biology-iv/respiration-animals/gaseous-exchange.php

The Importance of Citrates in the Kreb's Energy Cycle.
http://www.wiley.com/college/pratt/0471393878/student/animations/citric_acid_cycle/index.html

A S Silva et al, *Metabolic Acidosis, Sodium Bicarbonate and Sodium Carbonate.* Journal of Cancer Research.
http://cancerres.aacrjournals.org/content/69/6/2677.short

A S Silva et al, *The Potential Role of Buffers Reducing Intratumoral Extracellular pH and Acid Mediated Invasion.* Journal of Cancer Research.
http://cancerres.aacrjournals.org/content/69/6/2677.short

G F Filley et al, *Carbicarb, a Useful Ion-Generating Alkalizing Agent.* American Clinical and Climatological Assoc. 1985; 96: 141–153.
http://www.ncbi.nlm.nih.gov/pmc/articles/PMC2279642/?tool=pmcentrez

J H Sun et al, *Carbicarb, an Effective Substitute for Sodium Bicarbonate in Treating Acidosis?* PubMed Research.
http://www.ncbi.nlm.nih.gov/pubmed/2823406

B L Minton, *Balance Sodium with Potassium for Good Health.* Natural News.
http://www.naturalnews.com/024539_potassium_sodium_blood.html

S Disthabanchong et al, *Oral Sodium Bicarbonate Improves Thyroid Function.* Am J Nephrology.
http://www.ncbi.nlm.nih.gov/pubmed/21042013

A Rossier et al, *Sodium Bicarbonate Slows Progression of Chronic Kidney Disease.* Review Med Suisse.
http://www.ncbi.nlm.nih.gov/pubmed/21462516

R Caudarella et al, *Urinary Citrate and Renal Stone Disease.* Arch Ital Urol Androl.
http://www.ncbi.nlm.nih.gov/pubmed/19911682

Y Lu et al, *Citrates Induce Apoptic Cell Death in Gastric Carcinoma.* Anti-Cancer Res.
http://www.ncbi.nlm.nih.gov/pubmed/21498699

The Health Benefits of Sea Salt. Helium w/s.
http://www.helium.com/items/1870604-benefits-of-sea-salt

Mayo Clinic's View on Sea Salt. (*A completely inadequate view and understanding of sea salt.* Ed. note)
http://www.mayoclinic.com/health/sea-salt/AN01142

Epidemiological studies on the relationship between magnesium intake and heart disease. Magnesium Online Library.
http://www.mgwater.com/estudies.shtml

R Newham, *Boron the neglected element essential for sustainable healthy bones and joints.*
http://www.rexnewnhamarthritiseducation.com/paper.asp

Miscellaneous Articles and Research

GAO Report: Fragmentation and Inefficiencies of the FDA and USDA Agencies (2011). Food Safety News.
http://www.foodsafetynews.com/2011/03/call-for-one-food-safety-agency-leads-historic-gao-report/

M Louton, *The Real FDA Policy on Drugs.* Interview with Vioxx whistleblower David Graham. Natural News.
http://www.naturalnews.com/011401.html

Historic Lawsuit: FDA Sued Over Antibiotics in Farm Animals. Mercola w/s.
http://blogs.mercola.com/sites/vitalvotes/archive/2011/05/31/
historic-lawsuit-fda-sued-over-antibiotics-allowed-in-farm-animals.aspx

S Hamilton, *Criticisms of the FDA.* eHow w/s.
http://www.ehow.com/info_8514476_criticisms-fda.html

R E Laibow, *CODEX Will Destroy Our Nutritional Supplements and Organic Foods!*
http://www.healthfreedomusa.org/docs/codex_flyer.pdf

M Enig, *The Oiling of America.* Coconut Oil Research.
http://coconutoil.com/oiling_america.htm

M Enig, *A New Look at Coconut Oil.* Weston Price w/s.
http://www.westonaprice.org/know-your-fats/541-new-look-at-coconut-oil

C S Dayrit, *Coconut Oil in Health and Disease: Monolaurin's Potential as Cure for HIV/AIDS.*
http://acudoc.com/Coconut%20oil%20study2.pdf

C E Isaacs et al, *Inactivation of enveloped viruses in human bodily fluids by purified lipids.*
http://ukpmc.ac.uk/abstract/MED/8030973

L Ling et al, *Inhibition of Listeria monocytogenes by monoacylglycerols synthesized from coconut oil and milkfat by lipase-catalyzed glycerolysis.*
http://pubs.acs.org/doi/abs/10.1021/jf00030a033

D Harman et al, *Vegetable Oils, Aging and Cancer* (1957).
http://www.diabetes-diet.org.uk/unhealthy-fats.html

M L Pearce et al, *Incidence of cancer in men on a diet high in polyunsaturated fats (1971).* The Lancet.
http://www.thelancet.com/journals/lancet/article/PIIS0140-6736(71)91086-5/abstract

J Hull, Aspartame *Side-Effects*. Dr J Hull's w/s.
http://www.sweetpoison.com/aspartame-side-effects.html

R Blaylock, *Scientific Abuse in Migraine/Headache Research Related to MSG, Aspartame and Excitotoxins: The Taste That Kills*.
http://www.life-enthusiast.com/index/Articles/Blaylock

C Schubert, *Aspartame linked to increased cancer risk in rats. Nature Journal*.
http://www.nature.com/news/2005/051118/full/news051114-15.html

B S Reddy, *Dietary Fat and Colon Cancer: Animal model studies*. Lipids Journal.
http://www.springerlink.com/content/x0243w641u7q604n/

M Sircus, *The Poisoning of America's Water Supplies*. Natural News.
http://www.naturalnews.com/023565_water_lead_drinking.html

Global Agricultural Water Pollution. FAO Report.
http://www.fao.org/docrep/W2598E/w2598e04.htm

D R Davies, *Declining Fruit and Vegetable Nutrient Composition: What is the Evidence? Bio-Communication Research Institute, Texas University*
http://depthome.brooklyn.cuny.edu/anthro/faculty/mitrovic/davis_2009_food_nutrient.pdf

D Veracity, *Wheat and the Alloxan-Diabetes Connection*. Natural News.
http://www.naturalnews.com/008191.html

C Rose & P Gyorgy, *The Relationship of Dietary Factors to the Toxicity of Alloxan*. Dept of Gastro-Intestinology, School of Med., Penn. University.
http://jn.nutrition.org/content/39/4/529.full.pdf

Obesity and the Importance of Calcium/Magnesium Balance in Women. Obesity Research. Nature Journal (2004).
http://www.nature.com/oby/journal/v12/n11/full/oby2004229a.html

M Adams, *HFCS contains Mercury and other Chemical Poisons*. Natural News article.
http://www.naturalnews.com/032948_high_fructose_corn_syrup_glutaraldehyde.html

W C Leibhardt, *The Agricultural Agenda*. Agri. Research, UCLA.
http://hortsci.ashspublications.org/cgi/reprint/25/5/506?maxtoshow=&hits=10&RESULTFORMAT=&fulltext=poison+pesticides+&andorexactfulltext=and&searchid=1&FIRSTINDEX=0&sortspec=relevance&resourcetype=HWCIT

Dr Gerard Judd PhD. *Letter to the US Government on Fluoride and Teeth Health (2002)*.
http://www.life-enthusiast.com/index/Products/Dental/Dental_Health_Letter_to_Government/1

D W Miller, *Fluoride Follies*. Iodine4health w/s.
http://www.iodine4health.com/special/halogens/miller_halogens.htm

CDC and ADA Now Advise to Avoid Using Fluoride (2010). Mercola w/s.
http://articles.mercola.com/sites/articles/archive/2010/11/13/cdc-and-ada-now-advise-to-avoid-using-fluoride.aspx

G E Abraham, *Iodine Supplementation markedly increases urinary excretion of Fluoride and Bromide*.
http://www.iodine4health.com/special/halogens/abraham_halogens.htm

Background Books

Alkalizing Revolution by Vadim Guchinskiy: Createspace, 2010.
http://www.amazon.com/Alkalizing-Revolution-Vadim-Guchinskiy/dp/1451528043/ref=sr_1_2?s=books&ie=UTF8&qid=1310021812&sr=1-2

Alkalize or Die by Theodore A. Baroody: Eclectic Publishing, 1991.
http://www.amazon.com/Alkalize-Die-Superior-Through-Alkaline-Acid/dp/0961959533/ref=sr_1_1?s=books&ie=UTF8&qid=131002
3967&sr=1-1

Silent Spring by Rachel Carson: Houghton Mifflin, 1962.
http://www.amazon.com/Silent-Spring-Rachel-Carson/
dp/0618249060/ref=sr_1_1?s=books&ie=UTF8&qid=1345722566
&sr=1-1&keywords=silent+spring

ABOUT THE AUTHORS

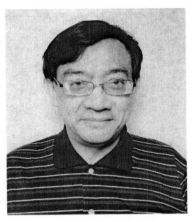

Parhatsathid Napatalung (AKA Ted)
Since 2003, Parhatsathid Napatalung
has been the preeminent expert voice
on integrative medical therapies for the
EarthClinic.com website, as that site
has grown from random blog entry
to one of the world's Top Two sites
on alternative medicine. The eager
and sustained interest Mr. Napatalung
draws to his continuing research into alternative and complementary
therapies for everything from mange in dogs to suppressing the
growth of brain tumors has played a central role in the website's
success, but that is nothing to the number of grateful readers who
commend his as the one voice that was able to save them from
debilitating illness when the rest of the medical profession had failed
or given up. With justifiable fondness and esteem, we have come to
know Mr. Napatalung more simply as "Ted" from Bangkok.

Ted was born in Bangkok, Thailand and has since returned to
that historic metropolis but spent the formative years of his life
(1965-1981) in the US, studying in its schools and universities. He
is an autodidact in the areas of biochemistry, allopathic medicine,
laboratory science, and integrative medicine as the outgrowth of a
very personal interest in life-saving treatments standard medicine has
ignored or missed out on entirely.

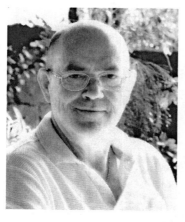

Bill Thompson
Bill Thompson entered the Earth Clinic community years ago as one of the walking unwell but has emerged not only wholly well but furthermore as an expert in alternative therapies. In particular, Mr. Thompson has established an eager following for his advice on alkalizing techniques and the treatment of systemic candida—two areas of complementary healthcare he has studied extensively and in successful application to his own health.

After a productive career as a software analyst and entrepreneur, Bill Thompson was able to enter into an early retirement in the Philippines, where he could launch into this second lifetime in alternative health. The analytical skills required by his first career and life-long interest in natural herbal therapies have made him the perfect counselor to weigh the evidence both for and against powerful natural remedies, and to present them cogently to a world of people eager for inexpensive, natural medicines.
Mr. Thompson, now in his sixties, enjoys the company of his family and the successes of his two grown sons.